SEIZURE

by

Joshua Holmes

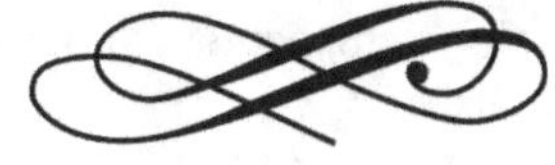

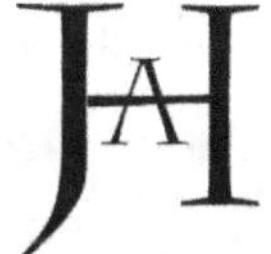

Visit Joshua A. Holmes at www.behance.net/Artman706

Printed in the United States of America

First Edition: Dec 2014

10 9 8 7 6 5 4 3 2 1

ISBN: 9798344913490

Imprint: Independently published

Library of Congress Control Number: 2014907742

CreateSpace Independent Publishing Platform, North Charleston, SC

Cover Design by Joshua A. Holmes

DEDICATIONS

This book is dedicated to my
Parents and Grandparents

AUTHOR'S NOTE

JUST A quick note to my readers: I loosely based this novella on my early post-collegiate experience. While I visited several of the described places, the characters aren't real and the expressed philosophies and worldviews aren't necessarily all mine. For the most part, this is fictional.

That said, the seizures I describe and the feelings and scenarios associated with them are real. I have to cope with them regularly, and I wanted my reader to better understand what persons with Epilepsy deal with, and ultimately to see what we are capable of.

As with everything in life, nothing stays the same. One could say I'm being redundant in my subject exploration, but the truth of the matter is that seizures change and since I've had so many types, it only makes sense to describe the similarities and differences in a clearly stated way, if not to raise awareness then to provide some personal therapy as well. Thanks again for your support.
–Josh

PART ONE

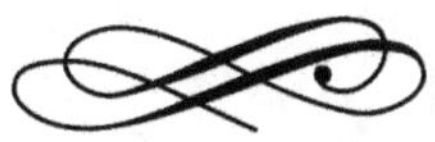

PROLOGUE
IN THE CAR

I FELL BACK towards him even though he kept push-
ing my body away. Over and over I tilted left, towards the
cup holder, the driver's side, only to reverse tilt a second
later, precipitating more shoves. I shook until my body
was a dead weight again, motor skills gone for now, but
I fought it. And so did he. One hand on the steering wheel,
the other, to an extent, hoisting my body up, he was afraid and
I was afraid.

I'd normally respond positively to the mechanics of a
buckle, but the resistance of the seatbelt against my chest
and at my waist frightened me. I began to panic. There
was this delayed unconscious moment I've yet to figure
out when my brain recognized I was scared, and it some-

how sent me into an even deeper state of adrenaline-laced terror.

I frantically tugged at the seatbelt. Pulled hard. Yanked with all my might, no sense at all in my actions. I continued to yank, toiling obsessively without rationale.

I profusely apologized to him, sorry that he had to witness this mess that was me.I did this every time. Was my action driven by guilt?

"It's OK, Chris," he said. "I'm here."

My throat burned. It was raw from trying to fill my lungs, to catch my breath. My chest was full of phlegm. I coughed.

The car was still moving, on the highway. High beams coming from the opposite direction nearly blinded him, nearly blinded me. I could hear myself crying, panting, could vaguely see my reflection in the passenger window.

"Chris. You had a seizure."

I let out a cry. The black macadam raced towards us, and it felt the yellow double lines would come right through the windshield.

"I can't breathe."

"I know. I am going to pull over, okay?"

"I'm so hot."

Hand to my forehead, I pushed my brown hair aside, dabbed sweat from beneath my bangs, and wiped it on my jeans. I was exhausted.

I saw cars pass us. Some drivers laid on the horn. Others shook their heads in disgust. And others still offered nasty hand gestures.

"You want the fans toward you? Just let me pull over."

He turned the car off a nearby exit, and pulled into a gas station. We just sat there, together, and tried to gather ourselves as best we could, considering.

He turned the fans on the dashboard in my direction.

"I can't take this anymore," I said, leaning forward. In that moment, I honestly didn't think I could.

• • •

I
JUST ANOTHER PLACE

AT ANOTHER place, but in the same position, I deduced; a different time, I sensed, but in the same splayed trajectory. Like a man on the cross, my left hand lay near my head to be anchored. And on the opposite side, my right hand waited as well. On my back, even my legs were overlapped, and I frantically looked up and then side-to-side, trying to figure it all out. Lots of people. Frowning faces. Heads shaking. Whispering. Worrying.

I had to be in public. Subway? Starbucks? Each location very possible.

Green. All around its green. Pine counters. Pine tables. Pine floor mats. Employees in pine aprons. No yellow in the sign above me, just a female in a pine crown and pine stripes. Enough for me to decide I was at Starbucks.

A bulky lady hovered over me. "I am an EMT in Baltimore," she said. "He needs to stay still until the ambulance gets here."

I had to stay still? Not again. With a deep breath, I tried to hoist myself up onto my elbows, to look around and soak up more of my surroundings but exhaustion overcame me.

The bulky lady pointed at a woman with several whiny young children. "Please take your kids outside, ma'am."

Geesh, I thought. *Do they really have to make such a big deal out of me? Am I that scary?* I couldn't remember everything I did or didn't, whether or not I shook, but I found it hard to believe it warranted all this attention.

Stone, the manager, stood in his pine apron a few feet away, leaning on a broom stick, and asked, "Are you all right, Chris?"

"I'm ok. I had a seizure."

The bulky lady interrupted. "You sure did, honey. Lay down. You hit your head pretty hard, too."

I HAD HIT my head. That's what Bulky said anyway. For the life of me, though, I couldn't find a knot or a tender spot. I rubbed my skull as I thought about things and waited for the ambulance.

I looked at the floor to locate a point of impact. I thought perhaps I had left a visible mark, but I didn't see blood or a burnished tile.

I saw my black, leather computer bag a short distance away. My computer was in there. All my ideas. My contact information for my current clients. What I once used for graduate work in the counseling field, I now used to assist me with freelance graphic design. I couldn't lose my computer or anything on it, otherwise I could kiss next month's paycheck goodbye. When you are pinned on your back, however, it's hard to collect any belongings.

I was disappointed to see the fabric had been ripped, I assumed, from the fall. The outside netting that held my pens and pencils was torn from corner to corner. Beyond the tear, though, the bag seemed alright.

The bag reminded me why I had visited Starbucks that day. It wasn't even a week prior when a pastor had contacted me about designing the interior and exterior of a children's book. We agreed to meet at the coffee shop to discuss all the technicalities and the cost. I now recalled it had gone as planned and I had reached an agreement with him.

I was having a decent day, went on to call and tell a friend about my good fortune. In that moment, however, I started losing my speech, the dreaded pre-cursor. I tried to talk my way through it, heard my friend asking if I was okay, but the next thing I knew, I couldn't speak at all. I dropped my phone, turned sideways, and twisted hard to the right until I tipped back in my chair.

IT ALL could have ended as formulaically as most commercial movies do today, my story I mean, but then again, where's the reality in that? My story continues. I imagine if you are reading this, I didn't traumatize you enough the first time around, and you are back for more. Well don't fret, there's plenty to tell you. Honestly, friends, as far as my Epilepsy is concerned, I still have it and the condition still manifests itself in ways beyond the average person's active imagination.

I didn't change my name, Chris, either, since I've yet to hear that any such change would affect the attributes of my Epilepsy. I know it's not a name with a lot of gusto, but it will grow on you. As far as I know, I could be a Frank, Charlie, or Mo, and still have to endure the thrills of my diagnosis.

I hope you catch my dry tone when I speak of "thrills." It's anything but thrilling. Several years after my fall from a seizure into the ditch in State College, PA, however, I am again preparing myself for a wild night of "thrills." All I can do is be a little sarcastic about it.

In any case, today really did start like most others. Sorry if that sounds cliché. And I should clarify that it started like any other day after my graduation from PSU and design school, and following my decision to pursue an art and design profession.

It was the beginning of December, a nice holiday reminder although the rest of the world seemed to have started celebrating in October. My room was a little chillier than normal, but it felt nice to cuddle a bit longer before convincing myself to rise and dress.

I noticed my torso and neck ached as I put my shirt on, and the comforters on my bed were askew, indicators of a seizure-filled night I couldn't recall. After I finally gathered my things, I decided to head out into the world. I didn't foresee an ambulance visit.

CHRIS. CAN you walk?" Another big-boned woman asked, the local EMT I guessed.

I was shaky, no question. Shaky and weak. I rubbed my knees, and took another deep breath. I felt the cold, textured tiles underneath me. "I should be able to."

I looked for the woman's name tag. I was disoriented, but finally located it, there with her title. She offered me a hand and said, "My name's Sally."

"And I'm June." The second EMT, rosy in the cheeks and slightly beefier, offered me a hand too.

I thought I vaguely recognized them both from a previous occurrence at another venue. I hoped for this so that I might convince them to consider what had happened in my other instance, and, bottom line, to forget protocols that just didn't work.

All the green around me disappeared, the decorative air vents and overbearing, duo-tone wall mural, as I was pushed unbuckled out the door into the bitter cold and falling white snow.

June said, "I do remember you." And then she went on to take down personal information from my silver, medic alert bracelet, among other things.

Once strapped into the aluminum gurney, the two local EMTs lifted me into the back of the ambulance with relative ease. From my perch, I stared out the vehicle's rear at the snowdrift and waited.

For those who've never been in this position, I can only describe it as surreal. A person can only be objectified so much until he or she goes into a self-protective mode. I went there whenever I was forced to lay within these tight confines.

But I eventually had to answer all the questions on their medical forms, and they called the ER, even though I would have preferred to sign release of service forms and head home.

More bluntly, I would've preferred the old way—when I had a say in my medical affairs. Now they performed the medical "services" first—the electro-cardiogram, the blood sugar test, the blood pressure test, to name a few—and then put my rights in the hands of the doctor on call, only reminding me of the charges after the fact, if prompted.

I understood that the EMTs had to make a living, don't get me wrong, but the hospital visit was pointless, like most of them. Yet it was beyond my control.

You see, what happens is this: by the time I arrive at the Emergency Room, my body has recovered, which ties everyone's hands. That particular night, I was wheeled out into the bright, ER hallway, left to wait. I didn't even have an assigned room. I enlightened the doctors though. "My body hurts all over," I said to half a dozen different physicians. "But I'll survive. No tests please."

• • •

2
THE CALL

I DIDN'T KNOW how to respond the day I received the call. It was random and brought up a lot of emotions I didn't even realize were still there. I knew I had attempted to block things out, to push it down for self-preservation, but I guess the hurt had just been covered by something else and left to sit deep inside.

That particular phone ring startled me, too, because I had been intently focused on assembling one of my design projects. I think I had been simultaneously watching a Youtube tutorial on unique font combinations, Photoshop filters, or something like that, and a TV talk show, when I was jarred back to reality.

"It's me, Chris. Michael." My former best friend.

I muted the TV, was silent a minute, then said, "I know, Michael. Hi."

I hadn't talked to Michael, or his new wife, Linda, since the day they officially quit school, since they left my apartment, a semester prior to my graduation in Penn State.

They both chose not to attend my ceremony, and I hadn't been invited to their wedding. I mean, I did tell Michael I thought he was stupid for dropping out, regardless of whether or not he was in love, which didn't go over real well, but I wouldn't have been a good friend if I silently agreed with every emotional thought he had and didn't give him some logic to mull over.

And that cross tattoo he had inked onto his wrist? Such a permanent mark! I never gave him grief over it, but to this day, I shook my head at the thought. Perhaps a popular move back then, I wondered if he'd regret it later.

In any case, while I accepted his decisions, I didn't like how things happened, and how we all had moved on without addressing the divide that inevitably emerged.

While I knew Michael and Linda were philosophy lovers, I couldn't tell you if either of them used the area of study professionally. And I didn't know if they debated for leisure any longer. I hadn't inquired about job choices, their general life direction, or anything else for that matter, and I still ached in my gut too much to ask or say anything that surpassed surface chatter.

I turned off the TV, shut down my computer, disconnected it from my surge protector, and set it aside.

"I'm coming to York later this week, Chris," said Michael. "Thought I'd call you up. It's been a while."

I turned over onto my back, spread eagle on the mattress, taking in the news.

A while? To put it mildly, I thought. He hadn't talked to me in ages!

"It has been a while."

IT AMAZED me what came to mind on my back after I set the phone down. The color of Michael's hair: red if he hadn't changed it. His quip, "Back to the good life." Whether he still said it constantly as he rubbed his goatee. Whether he still cooked awesome-smelling pancakes and nasty-smelling curry, or if he changed these habits to appease Linda. Women do mold their men, after all.

My mind jumped to our childhood. How long we had been friends. Our afternoons in the back yard. Our innocent talks about everyday discoveries.

It then jumped to his scar—my scar too—and our brain surgeries. His success, my botched procedure. His seizure-free life, my seizure-filled life. But I moved on quickly.

I jumped to Penn State, to college; remembered how close we were, and how separated we became. How his relationship with Linda ruined everything. Made Michael dismiss logic and fear my condition like every-one else under the sun. How it ultimately made me stronger, but less inclined to socialize.

I WAS WAITING for the bus again, thinking about my response to Michael's call, how I could be a good host, if I should be one in the first place. Shuffling my cold feet on the narrow berm of Queen Street, just beyond Waters Road, I could vaguely see over the mounds of salted snow the back of the older house into which I had re-cently moved. The relatively small, surrounding commu-nity, the bright neon lights of Suburban Bowlerama, En-terprise Rent-a-car, the powder blue exterior of the next door TV station, Fox 43, and a lot of speeding cars, as well.

The Red Rabbit bus was late again, because it was almost impossible to keep a schedule with holiday traffic, I knew. It would normally bother me, but I was busy thinking about my options as it pertained to Michael's visit. I didn't doubt my ability to act as a disconnected tour guide. It was the required, one-on-one interaction that at one point came so easily to me.

If it were anyone else, I wouldn't think twice about the meeting. Bottom line, I know myself well enough to see that I was allowing my emotions to rule, and I needed to get over my hang-ups quickly if I was to offer any semblance of decency.

I'd heard so many pastors and motivational speakers talk about the immediate choice to remain imprisoned, or to move on after a life hurdle, and how the choice affected the future; Though perplexed by the teaching at times, I didn't doubt that it was true. In fact, just then, I thought that the philosophy would be applicable here, and would resolve my dilemma if I could only speedily put it into action.

I chuckled to myself because I realized I had considered an unlikely possibility: speedy decision-making. Never would I, Chris, be speedy. Ever. It was just not a part of me. Fortunately, no one saw my random snicker, and I stroked my goatee to hide my smile and manage my expression.

I then adjusted my computer bag on my shoulder, and leaned on my dominant leg. I sighed and looked eagerly up the road for the red bus. Michael and I had been long-time friends. How could I just let that go? It would temporarily ease my angst, but not for long. I would eventually feel guilty.

I grasped my red bus pass tightly, and stuffed my hand into my deep coat pocket. A half hour later, the heavy whoosh of bus breaks sounded. As I stepped into the bus and swiped my card, I decided to pray about my situation and do the logical thing: stop dwelling on what was, and take everything one day at a time. *Re-focus and push on*, I thought.

• • •

3
LOOKING BACK

ANYONE WHO knew me well would confirm that I did my best work when I was troubled. Not such an unusual claim since many artists and designers throughout history composed moody masterpieces via creativity and free expression during tumultuous times.

While the feelings of tumult that inspired me were personal, and only emerged on occasion, in my opinion, I used them productively to complete portrait and animal drawings in pastel, colored pencil, and digital software, and did so to earn some extra money.

Over the years I had accrued quite a collection that affirmed my talent, encouraged clients to seek my specific style, and made school a lot easier to complete, as I had images around which to conceptualize.

Upon acquiring an illustration job, I usually set garbage bags or old towels on the floor area near my small closet.From that closet, I pulled out my blue duffel bag and orange suitcase chock full of supplies I've also accumulated over the years, a piece of suede mat board, and set to work in the inspired zone.

This was a practice that went back to my late high school days. I spent hours in the dank basement, by myself in the empty space. Under the grey lighting, I pondered over a piece, next to my stockpile of supplies, talk radio in the background.

Between my personal and professional life concerns, my spike in public seizure frequency, and my former friend's upcoming visit, I had plenty of inspiration to rely upon.

I had drawn for such a long time that, unlike many artists who drew out of fear, I composed with confidence. I recognized that inspired place, and created when it was there. I didn't worry about achieving a likeness of my subject, because I knew I'd eventually get there, regardless of any flaws in the process. As an artist, all I had to capture was a likeness. The degree of desired realism was relative, depending on who looked at the reference, and, ultimately, on who paid.

It took years, but after completing design school, I reached a point where I trusted my own judgment. I hadn't done anything, artistically speaking, that warranted a spirit of self-distrust, and in my mind, that was a major accomplishment.

LOOKING BACK, I accomplished a lot this year. I mean I try my best to succeed every year in everything I do; and to overcome my failures with other accomplishments. But this year, specifically, was a productive one.

Not everyone can say they graduated from Penn State followed by design school with honors and worked independently in the same field of study. I understand, however, the difference between doing several temporary projects, and building a client base for future projects and sustained business growth. My aim this year was to endure.

Like anything else, independent work had its challenges, the unpredictability for instance, but, so far, it seemed freelance design also had its perks: it suited my personality and presented an obtainable opportunity as far as making a living was concerned. I tried to keep it all in perspective, that life happened in stages, and experiences and opportunities came in waves, either temporarily knocking me down or surprising me with a new avenue to pursue. Sometimes I accepted it; other times, I struggled to. In any case, I can't endure too many of these platitudes, but can say that I'm interested to see what happens this upcoming year.

When there were opportunity droughts this past year, I took it upon myself to expand my knowledge base. It didn't take long—well, several interview rejections over a period of months, actually—to see that employers wanted graphic designers with web literacy. I took business and online courses in web coding and development: HTML, CSS, PHP, and JavaScript. While I did grasp the languages and design a website, I had more success in image manipulation, logo design, and corporate identity, and even more success in my lifelong specialty, illustration.

In my view, it just goes to show that we as humans are meant to find our talents, the gifts about which we are passionate, and pursue them either personally or professionally.

THE PASTOR seemed to agree with me the day we met at Starbucks. I shared my sentiments about using personal gifts, a little of my life story to break the ice, and he thanked me for being so open. He told me of the small church he led, of the pride he felt for the growing congregation, of the direction he wanted to see the church go, and made some general inquiries about my spiritual state and church attendance before moving onto our project.

"So tell me about your idea," I prompted that day. "Where I come into play . . ."

The pastor was a thin man; not Fed-Ex guy skinny, but not wrestler-heavy either. He smiled constantly as he sipped on his coffee. Took his time, too.

"Well, Chris." Slow sip. "I need an illustrator."

My ears perked up at the sound of a job. It was my area of expertise. I bit into a chocolate chip cookie, thought, Amen brother!

"And what do you need illustrated?" I asked, more personally than a car salesman, but less than a shrink. "It's a special ministry opportunity, actually Chris."

He went on to slowly describe his idea, to tell me of a story he wanted to develop, not unlike many that other of my clients had before.

"A ministry for kids," he added.

I briefly brought out a drawing pad and my laptop, and showed my skills. "I can illustrate something for kids on paper first, then use the Adobe Suite, and design anything else you might need."

"I know you can." His smile broadened. I sensed he was confident in me, and it did feel good.

"Any typographic preferences?" I probed. "Font families that you like?"

"Just pick something fun." I nodded and told him I could do that too.

We talked about my fee, and shook on it minutes later.

I was excited because I had used some of my counseling skills, built rapport with a potential long-term client, and done so on my terms.

I intended to lie on my bed as long as necessary, to conceptualize, and design in front of my Mac for many, many hours to help fulfill the pastor's dream and earn my compensation.

• • •

4
NEVER FORGOT HER

MARY GRACE'S presence was one that I never forgot, or even tried to for that matter. And I think the reason was two-fold: 1) she had always been the girl who made me feel special whether in grade school, high school, in college, or afterward, and 2) as a nurse at my current neurology clinic, she epitomized everything wonderful the rest of the nurse triage wasn't to me.

She made the appointments bearable. We both knew each visit would go the same way, bogged down by doctoral egotism, intrusive government procedures, and ultimately impacted by the most recent Epilepsy drug recommendations, which I always declined.

We both would later laugh about all the ludicrous side effects that came with the recommendations, how the doctors listed them matter-of-factly, commercial-like, and then justified them by saying,   "The company says it only happens to two percent." As if I'd never been that two percent before. And then how the staff looked in my direction, waiting for me to say, "Sure thing doc, can't wait for the blue fingernails, double vision, possible blindness, and, if I'm lucky, constant weariness."

Mary Grace always looked at me kindly from behind the doctor, with genuine empathy like she used to in the grade school gym, or high school football stands when I was upset I couldn't participate in sports, and her eyes just said, "Let it go." And I usually could.

I was beyond that idyllic association I once had, the notion that she was angelic and had a halo in my mind's eye, but I wasn't above saying that she was different, that she was in a class of her own, and that she left a lasting impression.

Since she gave me a nice check up, accepted my graduation ceremony invite, and attended the event, I had thought a lot about her, whether she had hidden baggage, whether she dated, whether she had kids, whether she thought about me.

I also said to myself, "Well, Chris, you invited her once ... why not do it again?" And I debated the question, always debating in my head.

One day, I'd work up the nerve.

• • •

5
CONCENTRATION

UNTIL THEN, I had to concentrate on finding interested clients similar to the pastor. That's to say, clients with authenticity, with a confidence and strong sense of trust in me, perhaps clients with an urgency to achieve their dreams.

While the aforementioned customer type was ideal, at the end of the day, I was open to finding any client. I knew they wouldn't all be like the pastor, which made each opportunity unique.

There were so many design opportunities out there, but twice, if not triple, the number of designers. And there was always someone better. I had to set myself apart, apply the standard marketing strategy of service/ product positioning. I had to find that one angle that nobody had yet approached.

I was different in that I had knowledge in other areas of study, English and Counseling, but in our current economy this fact seemed more of a detriment than anything, seemed to make employers think twice, to question why I hadn't gone further.

One thing I observed in school, though, was that students were either good or bad writers. Students were both fluid and poetic with their concepts and taglines, or they just missed the mark entirely. I happened to excel in the English area, and I made it a goal to offer editing and manuscript compilation services in addition to book cover design whenever I could. It wasn't necessarily unique to me, but it was a necessity for those who wanted to preserve the standards of traditional publishing, and no one in my immediate network followed suit.

I had considered taking it a step further, investing in my own website, postcards, newspaper and online banner ads. My electronic portfolio was substantial and had received plenty of notice, but it, too, could use an update.

I wasn't naïve, however. I was aware that, regardless of my positioning, of my ads, I had to re-visit my interview approach. It was complicated, I knew—so many factors at play—but a wrinkle that in time God would iron out.

• • •

6
EXTRA MEASURES

Every now and again, when there was a lull in freelance work, I would contact my design school to see if they had any job leads. I had started visiting the Career

Services office weeks before graduation to test the touted hundred percent job placement rating, and I never let up until I started pulling in my own clients with regularity.

I worked with a woman named Terrence Pincher. She was a spunky, trim, dark-haired lady in her fifties, I guessed, and her approachable air was perfect for the role. Her demeanor was engaging, and her raspy voice and throaty intonation was infectious.

I had called her a lot, initially. Probably more than I could recall. The early bird caught the worm, right? Why my peers never seemed to grasp this concept always amazed me, but their inactivity really did work to my advantage. And I wasn't surprised when she bellowed a loud, "Why hello there, Chris! What can I do for you?"

"Hi Terrence. How are you? Just calling to see if you had any freelance work for me."

"Doing well, here." A pause. "Actually Chris, I think I do."

"Awesome. Thanks so much."

"Let me see here. I have a name and number around somewhere." She let out a laugh as she rustled through her files.

I asked her what was going on at the school, if the annual portfolio show had gone well. Her answer usually told me whether or not it was a good time to call.

Aside from the graduation ceremony, the show was the pinnacle moment of the semester for Terrence, which required a lot of her time and energy.

"Oh the show went splendidly . . . a good turn out. And things are settling down now, so I have a few minutes to chat."

"Well I have a pen here, whenever you are ready." Terrence had several other graduates for whose employment status she was responsible, so I was glad to get her attention.

She gave me a number to a potential employer, explained that he wanted to grow his start-up and expressed interest in someone like me. I wrote it all down, excited for the opportunity.

• • •

7
PREPARATION

IT OCCURRED to me that I had two options for Michael as it related to sleeping at my place, and the second option was definitely more optimal for us both. He could either 1.) take my bed, while I took the couch—which tended to be uncomfortable—or 2.) I could stay in my own bed and room, and pick up a cheap inflatable mattress and charger at Bon Ton for my former best friend.

I didn't see the need to present the options, as I really wanted to sleep in my own bed, and I imagined Michael would prefer his own sleeping station.

There were places, I knew, that rented the noted items, but I was leery of that sort of thing, as I associated a rental with last resorts, and I wouldn't own the items for future use.

A Queensgate Plaza regular, I stopped by the strip mall Bon Ton on a mission shortly after, and thoroughly searched the premises for a reasonable, blow-up bed and battery charger. While the store never had applied a solid marketing and sales strategy, I occasionally found a deal hidden underneath the misleading signage.

I searched carefully, more quickly than I would elsewhere too, as the store was plastered in fluorescent lights, which often triggered seizures. I was sensitive to the brightness, and always had been.

I recalled when, back in the day, the chain had been one of the upscale types, and how it had later changed. Over the years, this particular store turned into an unusual hybrid of low-end and renowned products and clotheslines catered to the local neighborhoods. It primarily relied on overstock sales and coupons, and yet it remained open and relatively busy.

I often wondered how much longer it would survive. So many other stores had either closed their doors or gone bankrupt under the current administration.

In any case, I hated to part with eighty bucks, fifty for the mattress, thirty for the charger, but it was a need, and I would be able to use them more than once.

Upon arriving home, I unfolded the bed and uncapped the plug, tested the charger, loud and slow though it was, and a couple hours later, pushed the mattress against the wall at the end of my own bed.

Sleeping arrangements were settled. I now had one less thing to be concerned about.

PEOPLE DIDN'T seem to understand that, following a seizure in a public place, the person with Epilepsy had to ponder at home what happened, over and over, and muster the courage to go back to the place where they felt powerless and a sense of shame.

And to complicate matters, while he or she knew that the situation required attention, it was unwanted, and would most likely precipitate a change in how people treated them.

I didn't make this up. Even the ER nurse had given me a packet on the subject—which must have some merit—before I gladly departed my hospital cell. For whatever reason, I kept the packet up on my bureau.

Nevertheless, I wrestled with the issue while wrestling with the inflatable mattress that, until I later mastered the process, was more of a deflatable mattress than anything.

As I finished up with the inflatable bed, I had an urge for coffee. But that involved me heading back into the world. Sounded rational, right? Except I relived the seizure repeatedly in my head, and if I had to go face Stone, the Starbucks manager again, or endure another incident, I was sure I would scream. I even considered just staying in.

I also knew, however, that staying in meant I was living life fearfully. And I wasn't about to adjust for fear. I had done it too often in the past, and I was stronger now.

People asked me if my embarrassment was a matter of misperception. I despised that word so much. It was a politician's term. A relativist's term. In this context, though, perhaps it was a relevant point. And yet individual perception, in my view, was a person's reality, my reality.

● ● ●

8
FEARS CONFIRMED

STONE DID in fact confirm my fears. He treated me with a forced kindness I recognized from others who witnessed my seizures. When I re-entered Starbucks, again leaning on a broom in a green apron, he shouted, "Hey there, buddy! What can I get for you today?" Everybody turned and looked in my direction. I wanted to cower. The greeting wasn't that extreme, but it was different enough that it felt insincere and unnatural.

He could have been nasty or totally ignored me, and that would have felt worse, so I had to give him that much. Plenty of people had given me the cold shoulder after a seizure. I know everybody copes differently, but often it forced me to affirm people that I was fine, when, in actuality, I was in recovery.

Even now, it was hard to believe I was on the floor under the air vents and duo-tone mural a week prior. On the cold floor, shaking in the dirt. I had difficulty accepting it.

And there was no way that thought wasn't running through Stone's mind, as well. Even the best of feigners would fail to convince me otherwise.

"I'd like a Java chip Frappuccino," I said. "A venti, please." Stone, who was never previously an emphatic person, nodded his shiny, bald head with an exuberance that just didn't fit the request. I thought, *Way to overcompensate, there, Stone.*

"We have a special, today, buddy. A buy one, get one free, if you are interested."

I wasn't about to pass up a special, even if I got it on account of my disability. My take on it was this: if people felt better about the situation by gifting me with specials, I wasn't going to turn them down. I'm sensitive like that.

"Sure," I said. "Thank you. Sounds good."

• • •

9
EMERGENCE

STRANGE AS it might sound, the knot that I was certain would emerge on my head in fact never did. Delayed though it was, however, a week after my seizure, a piercing muscle spasm overcame my right shoulder, and proceeded to shoot bullets of pain into my mid-to-lower back and the base of my skull.

At first, I didn't consider it anything beyond another severe injury. But, as the days passed, I worried I might get addicted to the phone-prescribed pain pills. The spasms dulled with heavy muscle relaxants only to flare up again. I started to grow restless. The stabs were distracting and wouldn't stop nagging me.

Because I had sensory issues in my right side, the jolts were hard to settle and difficult to explain. I imagined they were akin to a wounded soldier's phantom pains and remember later contradicting myself when I said, "It's like a dull ache with sharp jabs."

As I went about my business, though, I noticed it was affecting my mood, and, in general, I just didn't want to be around anyone. I hurt too badly. Yet I knew I had to do something to alleviate the severity of my acquired injury.

So I attempted to consult with my neurologist, only to be put on hold when the nurse triage was preoccupied, and later referred to my primary doctor for reasons I've yet to find out.

After struggling to get solid answers from the specialists, I made an appointment with my primary doctor, and I crossed my fingers that I would leave the office with a legitimate treatment plan or credible diagnosis (although my Grandmother already diagnosed me with a concussion, as she had accurately done so often before).

* * *

10
HELPING

IN THE past, I'd been counseled to help others to keep perspective, told that it would solve my personal plagues. I tried it, and it didn't. Once I assisted at the YMCA. Another time I helped the church feed the poor. Did it take my mind off myself? Temporarily, yes. And did I feel a joy in helping others? Sure. Until, against my will, I was a public spectacle. And it happened more often than not.

I wanted with all my heart for the mere act of helping someone else to place all focus elsewhere. I wanted a random moment assisting an elderly person enter a church to resolve my pain problem.

Keeping focus was always a noble pursuit. At one time, I'd also been advised not to get distracted, that it was important to keep my eye on the prize.

At the same time, I knew the very fact that I wanted to help in order to overcome a crippling ache was a selfish desire, and couldn't be justified.

That was the catch-22 with the pain attack. So often, I had heard the clichés about mind over matter, how I could decide whether or not it would dictate the course of my life. It called to mind some of these extreme reality shows that demanded unrealistic living standards in the worst possible conditions.

I seemed to be losing the battle.

• • •

11
TECHNOLOGY BENEFITS

I NEVER THOUGHT I'd be one of these smart phone guys. But, as a confessed convert, I admit that once you leave dumb phones behind, there's no going back. Long time Apple fanatic though I might be, I hadn't expected to enjoy the upgraded cell's ease of use to the extent that I have.

And, believe it or not, it had nothing to do with the TV ads playing the latest pop hit in the background, exhibiting a one-word tagline noting the simplicity of the latest and greatest features.

For me, it was the visual experience: the colorful display, the streamlined apps, the organization that it provided. When the green voicemail app boasted a message it always excited me; made me wonder who wanted to speak with me.

Upon hearing the message, an inquiry from Mary Grace on behalf of the neurology clinic, I thought of her sitting there in a hallway chair, by the phone on the wall, the cord bouncing as she tugged the receiver, file cabinets and scale not far away. I was surprised to an extent: surprised by the immediacy of the call, but not surprised that it was my favorite nurse making the call.

"Hello Chris," she said over the phone. "I was sorry to hear you hurt yourself. Calling to check on the status of your head and neck injuries. Do me a favor and call the office. Ask for me."

I couldn't help but smile to myself. She cared enough to check on me. My expression would have been different, sour probably, if the other triage nurses had called.

I knew Mary Grace was doing her job; that she was following up. But I couldn't recall the last time a doctor or nurse reached out to me. I was always the one making contact attempts.

Mary Grace never ceased to amaze me.

• • •

12
REVELATION

AFTER THE Late Night Show with Jay Leno, one of his final monologues, I turned off the TV, pulled my covers to my chin, and closed my eyes to clear my head and pray. I talked to God for awhile. Afterward, I assessed what I had accomplished since mid-2013, a mental inventory if you will. What could I do to improve my situation? I wondered in the dark.

I was recalling what made me feel a sense of pride, what made me want to achieve a higher level of something, what made me invigorated.

Not to get super introspective or anything, but my mind wandered. I'm human. I thought about how I had spent so many years trying to please people; how it led to so much internal strain and emotional pain.

I even considered whether or not it was wise or healthy to go down that route, to think about such things since God pre-determined my path; whether or not I was exposing my mind to unnecessary stress.

Needless to say, my mind wouldn't stop.

I thought about my years studying karate, the few months Michael put in with me, the physical and mental challenge, performance-based and independent of opinion. Not my school studies. Not my design work. Karate.

It then occurred to me that, when studying karate, I also had pain issues, but the pursuit of physical and mental strength offset the battle wounds. It was pain with a purpose.

Here I was, in a latter life stage, trying to re-focus because the seizures and everything they entailed clouded my view, and it again hit me: I needed pain with a purpose.

• • •

13
PROCESSING

I DIDN'T THINK much more about Michael's random call in the next couple days or the blow-up mattress at the end of my bed because, before I knew it, his arrival time had come. I expected he would let me know when he made it to York. Until then, I'd make sure my place was suitable for a visit and try not to trip over the battery charger.

For so many years I watched my parents invest all their time and energy into hosting preparations for visiting family and friends, into carpet cleaning, bed making, into dinner planning, and so on. Admirable as it was, I wasn't about to put a bunch of money out for Michael. I would provide him with the essentials. Perhaps I would feel more generous in the future.

I did have an extra set of blankets and sheets, and a spare pillow and pillowcase that I pulled from my small closet and placed at the end of the blow-up. It escaped me earlier, but it hit me before it was too late.

Each day, as I prepared, I processed Michael's call and our shared past, and it grew a little easier to accept. I didn't feel the weight that initially pressured me, the conflict that occupied my mind.

We hadn't talked about anything substantial on the phone. I wished I hadn't been so caught off guard. We could have closed our past and paved the way for his visit to come.

But I failed to ask what he might want to do while in York. I hadn't prompted him about the matter, and he hadn't offered any indications. Perhaps we could catch a bite or attend a movie. Time would tell.

The weather was definitely inclement. But having walked the campus terrain for so many years, and now the uneven, wooded hillside along the roads, I was used to it. And I imagined Michael would be too, since he had to walk Linda home in similar State College conditions, and now whenever they went out together. It shouldn't pose a barrier, but worst-case scenario, we'd stay inside.

• • •

14
STORMS

I HAD ALWAYS loved the sound of storms: the sprinkle and pounding of rain, the static in the air, and the sporadic claps of thunder that followed fissures of lightning.

I loved listening to the wind whip the tree branches just outside my bedroom windows over and over against the wooden panes, to the house creak under the force.

I loved how, psychologically speaking, the stormy sounds of York made me feel a sense of peace and safety. I'm not sure where that feeling originated, but it might explain why, for years, I fell asleep to a sound machine with dripping water as its primary noise cycle.

But when I couldn't make time for said sounds, similar noises that immersed the bowling alley were the next best things. I thought about this the day I walked over to Suburban Bowlerama to inquire about a league.

I was not optimistic about leagues because it was early in the year, and they always seemed to cost an arm and leg, but I was pleasantly surprised. I saw the familiar face of Marge, the owner's wife, behind the counter, and I decided to ask about any available programs.

I had noticed, coming in, that a program for retirees was in progress. The older participants didn't seem to have a care in the world. I so wanted to experience that degree of nonchalance, and hoped for good news, for a program geared to younger people.

"As a matter of fact, honey, we have one starting next week."

"Wonderful," I said, leaning forward. "Do you have any info I can take with me?"

"Right here, honey." She handed me a flyer with a signup form attached.

I filled out the details, detached them for Marge, thanked her as she took the form, and headed home.

W HEN I got home, I unfolded the flyer to check out the specifics of the league. It was a "Pizza, Beer, & Bowl" league that took place every Wednesday night at 9:15 PM. It didn't require any previous experience, was relatively cheap if you paid weekly or monthly, and it just seemed downright fun. I wouldn't have any alcohol, but I expected to eat a few pizza slices and down a few sodas in between strike attempts. I planned to get my money's worth.

I admit that I had no clue what I was getting into. For all I knew, I could walk into the sequel of The Big Lebowski, whatever that meant. Beyond a former roommate's claim that the movie was a bowling classic, I only knew it consisted of an impressive cast but, otherwise, was unfamiliar with the plot, so my experience could also be something entirely different.

As far as building a social life was concerned, however, it could only improve via the league. Aside from going out with a few long-time friends every so often, I had grown sedate, and this new membership opportunity was something that I looked forward to.

• • •

PART TWO

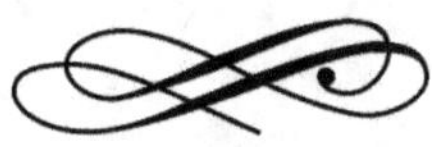

15
WAVELENGTHS

MURKY AND dark, my room was painted navy and adorned with long, floor-to-ceiling curtains that pushed away the falling snow's white hue, except for a narrow strip at the window's edge. I rubbed my achy neck as I pulled the curtains closer together. In that moment, it seemed the pain would never end.

Different wavelengths mess with my brain and my stubborn curtains were just then as well. I closed my eyes in a weak attempt to negate the pain and escape the two competing wavelengths, the darkness, the strip of light. I then opened my eyes when I realized I was just welcoming further spasms and light-induced nightmares.

"Please God," I said. "Spare me, please." For the millionth time, it felt, I was met with a silent, hollow noise.

I buttoned my pants in front of the window and rushed over to my pill container, hoping I could get my regular dosage in my system before the wavelengths messed with me any more and I had a big seizure. I lifted the container to my lips, but it was too late.

The pills missed my mouth and scattered all over the floor, under my bureau and bed skirt I guessed, but I was already busy thrusting my body onto my bed.

I thrust my body with aggression, with an almost illogical violence. I had to get onto the bed to keep me safe, I thought, regardless of whether or not it was injurious to my muscular or skeletal system. Once I reached mid-bed, I dragged myself even further up the mattress.

My strength waned quickly because I was cloaked in what felt like an unending pile of covers. Breathing heavily, I rolled to the left and right, crying out, fighting my constricted ribcage, my nearly paralyzed lungs.

Somewhere along the line, I lost consciousness, yet I continued fighting my body. I only know this because, once the incident was over, I came to on the ground, my muscles even more pulled than before. I was so exhausted that I just lay there, breathing and whimpering.

Eventually, I got up and again plopped on the bed. I drifted off a little. An hour later I decided to get going. I grasped the back of my orange recliner at my bedside, to gauge my balance even though it rocked under my weight and knocked the floor lamp behind it against the wall. I breathed.

• • •

16
GENERAL INQUIRIES

I WAS FORTUNATE that Mary Grace not only left a general inquiry message on my smart phone, but went on to kindly assist me when I called her back.

I casually observed the photo I had assigned to her number as we talked. I enjoyed her beautiful features: the light blue eyes, the high cheekbones and milky skin, the styled blonde hair that fell to her shoulders. And let's just say I had no difficulty remembering her curves below. She looked great, for sure, but it was more than that with her.

I didn't have to justify myself or prove to her that I was cognizant of my issues. So often, the other nurses would question the truth of my statements, as if I sat at home and made up stories about my seizures, as if I tried to create new symptoms or side effects to complicate their reports.

Perhaps other patients did this. I never really considered it before, but who's to say, with WebMD and the like available to everybody, that Hypochondriacs don't roam the net to seek proof for new conditions?

I briefly told Mary Grace of my most recent seizure, explained that I'd seen better days, but that I would survive, as I had proven repeatedly over the years.

"You are one tough guy," she said.

"I don't know about that, but thanks."

Mary Grace added, "We know you don't want any new meds, we know you aren't willing to try anything else, so we'll just go the non-medicinal route."

"This is why I love you Mary Grace," I ventured. "You are the only voice of reason in this place." I smiled.

She laughed. "So I will go ahead and send a prescription over to the local physical therapy office."

"For my neck, head, and shoulder."

"That's right," she added. "They should be able to help in ways we can't."

"Thanks so much, Mary Grace. It's nice to know someone is holding the fort down there."

$$\bullet \quad \bullet \quad \bullet$$

17
SPEED AND MASS

ALTHOUGH MARGE promised that, pending any seizures during league competition, no emergency calls would be made, I wanted my first night to be a smooth experience for everyone. The last thing I wanted was to scare my teammates and spend the rest of my time trying to convince them I was okay, or worse, thwarting alienation.

So, in order to familiarize myself with the environment, to dull the stimuli from the lights and speakers and crowds, I went over to the alley early.

As I walked through the front door I was hit with that leftover smell of cigarette smoke mixed with vacuum cleaner residue. Not a clean smell, but not a foul stench either; just a stale one. Recently turned smoke-free, the alley was far better than it used to be, but still musty and clingy as all get out.

I opted for the smell of grease, and for lunch had a grilled cheese meal with fries and an iced tea at the snack bar, followed by a coffee to wake me up. I sat back in my chair and watched a few die-hard bowlers practice their spins, no concern for the game's cost. I had a private physics lesson right then and there.

From what I gathered, achieving the proper thrust, or balance of speed and mass, was the key to a winning game. The lighter the ball, the faster the die-hard had to throw. The heavier the ball, the less he had to exert himself. It made perfect sense to me.

In the ensuing hours, the alley grew more and more congested. The smell of sweat started to mix with the cigarette, vacuum cleaner, and grease. I felt I adjusted well to the business and odors around me, though. I didn't have an increase in anxiety, lose my ability to speak, experience any auras in my eyes or bubbly sensations in my molars, so I was convinced my first league night would be safe and uneventful in a good way.

I SUCCUMBED TO my impulses that afternoon, bought a new black and gold bowling bag from the Pro Shop that would help the transit from home to alley, and identify my football team loyalties. It might even initiate conversation between my league mates and me.

I blamed the constant promos on the TV screens above the lanes advertising Pittsburgh Steelers paraphernalia. But I'm a sucker for sales, in any case, especially when the branding catches my eye. I justified the purchase by asking, "How often do you buy bowling accessories, Chris, really?"

I transferred my personal maroon, navy, and neon yellow-streaked bowling ball and white, Dexter bowling shoes over to my new bag, and, I had to admit, updates to belongings were nice every now and again. I felt better about myself that night, temporarily anyway.

I'D ALWAYS heard bowling was a blue-collar sport, which in my limited experience, meant it drew a different kind of crowd than I knew. This didn't concern me or anything, since I was looking for something different, but I did mentally prepare myself for any and all possibilities.

And there were a few teams who were definitely more rowdy than others, teams who liked to make a scene and messed with everyone else's head by utilizing the shock factor—yells and expletives at crucial points in the game. It also could have been the beer, I suppose.

But I was assigned to play with a reserved foot doctor and a well-spoken hulk of an ambulance chaser, who both were laid back, carried on good conversation, and also just happened to be amazing bowlers. I had to step back and give myself a pep talk about making premature judgments.

After surviving a harmless initiation prank—a practice throw on a closed lane—and a small scolding from Marge, I seemed to fit in almost immediately. They had a laugh at my expense, but I didn't react much, and I guess they appreciated that I could take their jabs.

I learned my lesson, though. I never tossed a pre-mature practice ball again.

So WHY feet?" I asked over soda and pizza that tasted like better than average, cafeteria food.

"No particular reason," the foot doctor, Burke, responded. "Why any field?"

"I don't know." I said. "I guess you could have helped old people or kids. I was just curious."

"Geriatrics?" Eye roll. "Pediatrics? You haven't given me many options, Chris."

My body still hurt from my seizure at home—especially my right shoulder and back region—so I sat back and enjoyed the talk, as trivial as it was.

"How about Neurology?" I asked.

"Foot pain is where the money is," Burke said to me.

"I can see that," I said. "I get those lifts for my shoes on occasion."

"If he's honest with you, Chris, he'll admit he wanted to specialize in Bunyan removal!" shouted Bender, the ambulance chaser.

The TV above our lane flashed the statement "15-minute practice starts now!" We wiped the grease off of our hands, and pulled out our individual bowling bags, balls, and necessary attire.

"Bunyan removal!" shouted Burke with a grin as he threw a strike. "Is that the best you can do, Bender?"

"I thought it was good," Bender shot back drily.

"Don't come crying to me, Bender, when you've hurt your feet running after a new case."

My BOWLING average was miserable, to put it mildly, by the end of our twenty frames, but Burke and Bender were nice about it. They both told me not to sweat it and my numbers could only go up from there. Little did they know.

"Get this strike, Chris," said Burke during my last frame. "And we'll do shots." I smiled, tried my best, and threw a wicked spin that missed a strike by inches.

"I'm doing shots anyway," said Bender. And he ran off to the bar.

In the next several weeks my abnormal bowling form would lead to consistent inconsistency and personal frustration. What can I say? I'm a perfectionist. My teammates were amazed by my imperfect stationary stance and my strong curve, but my position and throw inevitably tired me out before my fellow leaguers and kept me around 100 points when Burke and Bender doubled that. So much for the physics lesson.

"Almost had it," they would say. "We'll just hit above our average to offset your score. No problem."

I was glad that I had no seizures the first night, didn't even really have to talk about them, and that it was generally a decent opportunity to interact with some neat guys.

The casual nature of the league did help me to walk away, annoyed though I was at my performance. There was a hint of relief, a glimmer of hope that next week I'd improve my average and come through for the team.

• • •

18
CRUNCH

WHEN I heard the crunch of car wheels on the driveway the next morning, my heart started to race. Michael was here, and I was not ready. As I rolled over to put my glasses on and check my phone clock, I muttered, "Oh crap."

I hurriedly pushed my blue-striped covers back, sat up in the darkness, and rubbed my shoulder as I scanned the room for my clothes. My pants were on the floor in the usual place, and I had an assortment of t-shirts at the bottom of the bed.

I guessed he hadn't called me to announce his arrival like I thought he would because it was still morning, and he didn't want to disturb me. He could have forgotten, but I was inclined to give him the benefit of the doubt.

I heard the car door slam outside and the double beep of Michael's horn indicating he had just locked his vehicle. I imagined his walk to the house's side door, and tried to win an imaginary race, to dress, make my bed, oh, and can't forget this, take my medicine, before Michael knocked on the door.

The situation took me back to my college days, when on occasion I accidentally overslept the start of a morning class, and I rolled out of bed and ran, after taking my meds, dreading the inquiring eyes of classmates and the derogatory remarks about punctuality from bitter professors.

I presently threw my covers back into place, put on my pants, pulled on a golf cap, brushed my teeth, and ran to the side entrance just as I heard the first rap on the door.

I unlocked the doorknob and looked up to see a less fit version of my old friend. I noticed he was still a redhead, that he still had unshaven red facial hair. *He's obviously past the honeymoon phase of marriage*, I thought. And then I leaned out the door to see if Linda was around.

"Come on in, Michael."

"Thanks," he said. "And, by the way, Linda couldn't make it. But she says hi."

"I see."

"She did want to, but she had to work."

I picked up the suitcase that rested at his feet, and lugged it to my room, next to the blow-up mattress.

"We'll survive, I'm sure."

"Yes."

"To be honest with you, I usually dine out and relax at the coffee shops. The house is pretty barren, so if you want to stay in, we can watch TV or something. If you want to head out, though, we aren't far from numerous restaurants, two movie theaters, you name it.

"Well, let's get situated here, and then head out for lunch. I'm famished."

"Ok then," I said. "I am too."

THE LAST lunch we had together was at the Kern Graduate Building at Penn State Main. It was more of a relationship update on Linda and an apology from Michael for keeping me in the dark. So much time had passed. I had earned two collegiate degrees and done freelance work since.

Looking back, that update and apology should have sufficed. At the time, I believe it had. We even went from that sit-down and walked to North Atherton Street to check into the free karate lesson advertised and offered downtown.

I had always been assured that time heals, but in the next several months, I learned time can burn too. I was exposed to the harsh social reality of disability life: a person who was once loyal–Michael, for instance–would turn on me because I was different, perhaps even a threat to normalcy, whatever that was.

I had cleared my head by staying focused on my studies, on my art, and my martial arts routine.But Michael and Linda continued to push me away, altering my lifestyle, and the sincerity of Michael's initial apology was soon in question.

I wondered if Michael even remembered.

"Earth to Chris," I heard. "Snap. Snap."

"Sorry," I replied. "Was just thinking."

"So where are we headed, Chris?"

"Well you're driving, Michael, so it's your call. You know I'm terrible at split-second decisions. When it comes to food."

"Yes you are."

W E ATE at a place called Wonderful Gardens, a Chinese restaurant owned by a man and wife who cooked superb dishes, but who were a bit stingy with their service.

Like the exterior of Bon Ton across the street, there were days when it appeared dark and empty, and I questioned whether or not the place had gone under. ButI was glad to see the neon Open sign flashing in the window this day. I later noticed a door that led to an upstairs loft, where I imagined the couple lived—which meant they could open or close any time they wished, really.

The woman poured us both a cup of tea without a word, and left before we could order. Michael and I just kind of sat there chewing on the free prawn crackers.

We waited a while, ordered our meals eventually. Sometime later, my beef and broccoli arrived, and his General Tso's chicken came out shortly after.

The small talk we used to just ease right into seemed to evade us both. I remembered nights when we impersonated eclectic professors, when we sang random songs into pretend microphones and strummed on air guitars on the couch. It didn't appear we'd be concert-playing anytime soon.

"You like it?" I finally said above a tranquil, Asian version of a modern American radio ballad. It was definitely different from the all-you-can-eat Chinese buffet across town.

I kept the conversation light, told him this restaurant had been a family favorite for some years. We laughed a little about the mural on the wall of a near-naked sumo wrestler grinning smugly, it seemed, at the customers under his watch.

"Not bad," he replied. "Was so hungry, though, I could've eaten my fist."

I told him that if he wanted to do his thing that I could meet up with him later. Or if he wanted me to hang out with him, I could do that too.

"Yeah Chris. Good thinking," said Michael. "Let's meet back at the house tonight."

I was a bit surprised by his choice but a little relieved too. "Alright," I said.

• • •

19
ROUTINE

I SPENT THE afternoon at Starbucks. I know. You don't even have to think it. I frequent this place a lot. Could probably cut back, even. But its been built into my routine for quite some time now, and I happen to accomplish a lot with a computer and coffee in hand.

Call it a schedule, a routine, a focused action, an intentionality—as one pastor put it. In my usual recliner in the back, I had learned so many things, designed so many things, made so many contacts that it just made sense to work here. The results almost justified the money I put out for the ambiance, treats, and lattes.

Though Stone had treated me differently the last time I visited, with a sympathetic kindness I passionately disliked, I hoped for a genuine greeting, and thought he deserved the benefit of the doubt. He deserved another chance.

I was happy that he treated me like any other customer at the register. No specials just for me. He offered me a smile, said hello, asked what I wanted, and told me the barista would have my order out shortly.

I smiled and went my way. Was that so difficult, now, Stone? I thought to myself. Just keeping it real.

TERRENCE PINCHER, my career counselor, had given me that name and number to call for work, the man pursuing a successful start up, and I had yet to contact him.

I put my cell phone charger on the side table, leaned over and pulled my smart phone from my coat pocket. I called and an automated female voice instructed me to please wait. I would be helped momentarily.

The automated voice continued. She explained the startup was called Synergex, led by Rex Stealth, had been thriving for a number of years, that it was local and listed a number of accolades without stating exactly what they were about. And then there was silence.

As if on cue, Mr. Stealth broke the silence. He answered with a low voice that was half animated, half asleep. "Stealth here. How can I help you?"

"Hello Mr. Stealth. My name is Chris, and Ms. Pincher said you were in need of a designer. Just wanted to make contact and introduce myself."

"Well, tell you what. We are having interviews at the moment, and if you are willing, we could set up the first phone interview right now."

"Oh. Sure." Abrupt and to the point, but it worked for me. "You give me the time, I'll be ready."

We agreed on a morning call on a day the following week, and I thanked him for his time. I clicked off and put my stuff away. I had to get home to meet up with Michael.

BEFORE HEADING home, I ran by the physical and occupational rehabilitation facility Mary Grace had suggested. If I didn't check into it, I'd never know whether or not my pain could be controlled through this method.

The lobby was small, had just enough room for the six or seven waiting patients. One sat in a wheelchair, one sported a cast, and the rest appeared injury-free, although I knew they had something they needed to fix. I didn't have an overtly visible injury either.

I was glad that the lobby cleared out pretty fast. The facility accommodated quite a number of people at once, staff and patients, and it kept things moving efficiently.

When it was my turn, I was led to a back room and advised by a therapist named Val to fill out a pain assessment form, and to take off my sweatshirt so that she could massage my neck and shoulder, and follow up with an ultrasound.

I was in there for an hour—longer than I expected—and, boy, did I feel achy afterward. I was tight. I would remain so for several weeks until I saw my chiropractor in addition to my therapist.

• • •

20
RED EYES

MICHAEL'S EYES were red when I saw him that night. I noticed he was on the verge of tears at lunch, but I didn't think it necessary to mention. I didn't want him losing his composure in public.

"What's the matter?" I asked, surprised at my friend's display. "Why are you crying?"

"It's Linda, Chris."

"What about Linda?" I sat in a chair across from him.

"I lied to you. She didn't stay home because of work. She left me, Chris."He started crying pretty loudly right then. His shoulders shook as he cried.

"What do you mean she left you?"

"We got into a huge fight. We argued badly and she stormed out of the house."

I had known she was the diplomatic type, addressing issues politically—either via diversion or as an intermediary.

"Could she be at her parents' house?"

"I don't know. It's nearly been a week."

"What was the fight about?"

"Oh. It was something small initially. I didn't comment on her new haircut, and she took it to an entirely different level."

"New level?"

Michael started pacing. "She accused me of not caring about her anymore, of falling out of love, and so on and so forth."

"Which isn't true, right?"

"Definitely not!"

"And you don't think you are overreacting?"

"Overreacting!? No. I'm not overreacting!"

"It's worth asking."

• • •

21
KINKS

IT HAD to be frustrating for my physical therapists to work out the kinks in my neck and shoulder only to be informed that it's hard to tell whether or not there's been noticeable improvement because of my seizures.

I wasn't going to lie, though. It would defeat the purpose. While I was willing to admit that they had stopped the jabbing in my head and back, and isolated the pain to the neck and shoulder regions, the ache was still irritating and far from gone.

I had run into similar problems in the past. A seizure between treatments altered everything, and to pin a pain problem on one specific thing when so many muscles and bones were at play was a lost cause. I wouldn't be surprised if I said this again.

I'd almost forced the doctors and chiropractors and therapists to approach my body like an old car. When my parts cracked or when I stalled out, so to speak, I was either lubed up with meds, or gently coerced to turn over for massages, to get my engines going again.

So how is this any different than what other persons with disabilities go through? Only my friends with

Epilepsy can relate on the same level. An on-site observer might understand the required degree of determination to push ahead after experiencing an episode.

• • •

22
SOFT SKILLS

REX STEALTH did call me for a second phone interview, but spoke to me with the same level of interest he bestowed on me the first time around. I didn't understand why he even bothered if he didn't intend to hire me.

I went over my academic and professional background, and tried to explain what set me apart. He acknowledged my background, and moved on to other things.

Apparently, Synergex wanted specialists—individuals who didn't work beyond the scope of their specialty—and he wanted to make sure I understood this.

I was surprised because it wasn't many years ago when additional soft skills often made you a better, more qualified candidate in the job market. Now it over-qualified me!

By now, I had found his online profile, the company site that I was trying to improve, and all the additional staff—who just so happened to be family members. Rex sported a long mullet and every kind of non-traditional dress you could imagine. He expressed pride in nonconformity.

He spoke of casually assembling the existing site on a beach in the Caribbean, and of the fact that he knew it needed work. Perhaps I, if everyone agreed, would be the one to improve the Synergex marketing scheme.

I promised that I would do my best to offer up a feasible design option. He said he looked forward to seeing it.

• • •

23
TIME

MICHAEL'S DILEMMA made me think about time, the measurement of our lives, how he had messed up and just how much I could waste or produce, lose or gain, in a certain period.

Yes, I know, its an abstract line of thinking, but, having seizures, my sense of time alters with each episode, and what I can and can't do in a day or week depends on whether or not my body is functioning physically, or if I'm firing on all cylinders mentally, to use a cliché.

"Do you remember the way they felt?" I randomly asked, referring to Michael's seizures. "Or have you forgotten with time the sensations, the Postictal?"

If one looked up the term Postictal online, the site would loosely describe it as the near-hallucinatory state persons with Epilepsy experience just after a seizure. I was not sure that I totally agreed, but I guess it could vary from person to person.

"It was such a long time ago, dude, he said after a minute. "I sure didn't try to remember them."

"I was just curious," I said. "You know, I have a seizure, and then once it's all over, it seems days have passed, when its really only been a few hours."

"Yes. I know."

"On a different note . . . what are you gonna do about Linda?"

"I don't know."

"Well you aren't just going to let her walk out of your life, are you?"

"I suppose not."

"I don't mean to be rude, Michael, but I think it's about time you found Linda, and tried to make amends."

• • •

24
THE BETWEEN SPACE

IT WAS bound to happen, I thought. I had prayed I wouldn't seize there, but it definitely was a selfish prayer, and I'm pretty sure selfish prayers don't pull as much weight as those aligned with His will. And I was at the alley a lot.

In any case, I was in the small room that housed racks of mid-weight bowling balls when I took the headlong plunge. I barely missed the racks.

I had felt the seizure starting in the restroom, the fluorescents playing with my eyes, but had no time to react. No time to warn anyone. I didn't even have time to protect myself, to curl up in a fetal position for instance, as I had done many times while attend- ing school.

I stumbled forward, through the men's room door, managed a few steps, and then, somehow, twisted my way past the racks, into the group of bowlers sitting at the tall tables drinking beer and teasing each other about tournament scores.

I think the expressed horror, the shrieks, and the generally fearful reactions were heightened by the fact that I dreaded making a scene in a place that was my weekly source of entertainment. I couldn't bear the aftermath.

By now, you understand, from that point on, I was at the mercy of those who found me. Well intentioned or not, they determined the civility or lack thereof. It was no different that night.

THE BETWEEN SPACE is what I called it. The hellish period just after the seizure ended but before I was recovered. It was, in my opinion, the time when I felt most oppressed—confused, scared, exhausted, and out-of-control.

There was something about the alley, as well, that exacerbated the situation. The weight of my oppressive bout was ten times that of any I had previously endured. And it wouldn't end.

Just keeping my head up was tough. My body still dead, motor skills not yet returned, in the Between Space, a smile randomly plastered my face, although it was purely neurologic and definitely not indicative of my true feelings. My body tipped left and then right. Sometimes I landed without injury. Most of the time, I wasn't so lucky.

A doctor might say it was still Postictal, and perhaps some of my symptoms were, but take it from me, the people around me pushed me to the Between Space.

Think about it, my brain was just electrocuted and I was supposed to respond as if it was just another day?

On the one hand, you had the doting caretakers who sat with me, asked me questions, simple and direct yes under normal circumstances, but hard to answer when attempting to function in the Between Space. To complicate things, these caretakers, upon hearing a response often made near delirium, took what I said as normal communication, and asked the same questions over and over until my answer appeased their concerns.

On the other hand, you had the establishment leaders—owners, supervisors, managers, you name it—who made it clear they understood and believed me when I talked, but who, in actuality, were concerned about getting sued; liability their main focus. What got me the most, though, in the Between Space, was that they said, "It's nothing personal, just following procedure," as if, on top of coping with the physical exhaustion and mental strain, I should be able to deal emotionally too, no problem.

There was always that group of onlookers who talked about me and didn't know I knew what they were doing, and had no qualms about loitering over me, adding to my claustrophobia, while, inevitably, there was always one other person whose conscious made him step away and call 911.

AND IT still wouldn't end. Next I had to deal with the cops. Tall and barrel-chested, they drilled me much like a person who had just committed an offense. They even incorporated the stereotypical good guy-bad guy interview techniques.

"Come here, Chris. Listen up. I understand where you are coming from, but the doctor wants you to go in to the hospital."

"So that's it? I can't decline the doctor's orders?"

"No Chris."

"I just can't believe I have no choice." I turned away, so tired and livid, but out of options.

Simmons ended up on the scene, of course. The one cop I had nightmares about. Call it irony, a divine joke, take your pick, but he stomped over to the "scene of the crime", and took a shrine-like stance, as if his very presence demanded worship.

"You either go with us or in the ambulance," said Simmons. "We won't give you the treatment the EMTs will."

I gritted my teeth, shook my head, and clenched my fist at my side.

What was it with some officers? The posturing that took place was as much due to fear as it was ego. And, again, I understood they were human. But, it seemed, some- where along the line, they forgot that I was too.

"You can't put your officer persona aside a minute and just take me home? Its right across the street."

"No. I can't do that."

I'll just spare you my thoughts of the medical community. I crawled into the back of the ambulance. Went through their drill. Little by little, just as I had said would happen, I emerged out of the Between Space. By the time I was at the hospital, I told the doctors what would occur, and all three laughed at my procedural knowledge.

While the doctors laughed, I filed a grievance with my insurance company. I didn't see how improvements would occur if I remained silent, accepting the unacceptable, so I made sure my provider knew every oversight and act of misconduct.

I was sick to my stomach for days, it was so traumatizing, my experience in the Between Space. I dreamed about it repeatedly upon leaving the hospital. It eventually passed, however, after I told God I was shot and asked Him to calm me.

WHERE DID healthy self analysis end and destructive self obsession begin? Surely there was a happy medium. Yet I had pondered this for years, longing for an answer.

I asked this because, in that moment, at the hospital again, I knew something had to give: notably, how I, a single, middle-aged guy with Epilepsy, coped. I questioned everything, doubted a ton, until I was too exhausted to continue.

If I examined why anymore, or what was the cause of my condition, the reason behind my pain, and the subsequent events, I was bound to break. I was on the brink, so troubled by the seizure re-runs in my head, and the talks with God that didn't yield reciprocity, as I knew it (that's not to say it wasn't there, because I didn't sense it).

It was one thing to fall back daily on spiritual words of wisdom for consolation, or to use as reminders of what my verbal and active responses should be. It was another to actually apply them and comfortably accept them.

The discomfort of living in discomfort was maddening. Constantly wondering about the purposes of things I might never know was even worse.

If I was honest with myself, though, I had to decide right then and there if I could let everything go. Not just say it. But actually do it. And feel alright with it. And not just some of it, either. It couldn't work that way.

I hated that I had to experience the hell that I did, to the degree that I did, to reach this point, but isn't that so typical of the human experience?

· · ·

25
THE RETURN

I DIDN'T EXACTLY know what Michael expected from me. He'd obviously come to York to escape his relational shortcomings with Linda, and was using me as a convenient vacation.

Here I had spent all this time processing the moments he hurt me in college, and it turned out he needed the past to be the past, and wanted me to act as some kind of living tutorial.

Considering how I initially focused on his betrayal, I think Michael benefited most. I didn't torture him over the initial lie, and I feel I commiserated on an acceptable level without guilting him.

On two separate occasions I went on to pose reasonable questions regarding his current state, and even offered up some constructive analysis.

I hoped he didn't intend to stay for an extended period. While I wanted him to fix his problem, it ultimately wasn't up to me, it couldn't be resolved here, and had to be resolved there.

I understood the need to get things out of your system. But life had to move ahead. I only had so much room fora vacating, weepy adult.

And, I admit, if I haven't already, that helping Michael a few days had taken my mind off my pain and my seizures. I temporarily focused on getting Linda back. But it was temporary.

I was both surprised and happy to see—upon arriving home from the hospital—a letter from Michael. He must have sensed that I wanted to help, but also that I didn't want the visit to be long-term.

He wrote:

Chris —

Thanks for your hospitality.

You helped me realize what I lost and that I can still save it.

I've decided to go home and make amends with Linda.

Thanks,

Michael

● ● ●

PART THREE

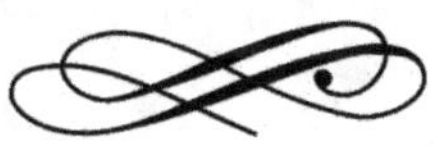

26
THE MISSION

I TIGHTENED MY schedule over the next couple of months, visiting the rehab facility twice a week, if not more, and stretching nightly before I went to bed. I didn't fill a calendar or anything, but my time was put to good use.

I had to fit my art and design projects in between the appointments, usually on the odd days of the week. We reached a point where we set back-to-back appointments to logistically accommodate me.

I even started eating at the next door grocery store—soup or fried chicken and tea at Weis Markets—so that I could accomplish multiple things on any given day.

On occasion, I even ran into one or two of the therapists who met their spouses for a quick meal over break, which made for a nice yet awkward greeting.

As I mentioned earlier, the discomfort in my head and shoulder would wane with each of the ultrasound treatments, only to return a couple days later. So I made it my mission to overcome the jolts of pain with repetitive exercises.

I became one of their regular fixtures. I got along with everyone, and we all were determined to regain my lost physical capacity. I'd do a half hour of stretching, and a half hour of strengthening.

The battle with my body continued for four months. My bowling game fluctuated, depending on the length of a treatment. I worried things might never improve, but my work and their work eventually paid off.

In the fourth month, the pain-free periods began to grow longer and longer, and my therapist hinted at the possibility of wrapping up my treatment sessions.

I noticed the improvement at the bowling alley, while relaxing at home, in my everyday transportation efforts, and, though I told them they'd miss me, I agreed things were better and could see they had to give my insurance company results.

• • •

27
TO CAVE OR NOT

I DISTINCTLY REMEMBER the night I had to decide whether or not it was worth continuing in the league. I must have changed my mind a good ten to fifteen times about walking over to the alley.

I was uptight and overheated, for one, and there really was no guarantee, as there never was, that the evening would be event-free.

I clearly identified my apprehension as a fear or phobia, and I knew the only way to defeat it was to place myself again in an uncomfortable spot.

I tried to question myself as objectively as I would have questioned a client in a counseling session, sparing nothing, so that I made solid decisions.

I had been forced to do this in numerous contexts—professionally and academically—throughout my life, and I surmised this would just be one more instance where I'd have to suck it up, and flush out the emotional wounds later.

I skipped practice and watched TV in my room until I could postpone play no longer.

I picked up my Pittsburgh Steelers bowling bag, put on my shoes and jacket, and made my way across the street. It's hard to explain, but even in that mentally strong moment, I felt emotionally raw. It took several weeks for that feeling to disappear.

WHAT HELPED me integrate back into the league culture so quickly was the fact that Burke and Bender never brought up the seizure. They no doubt had heard about it, no doubt knew I was pretending it hadn't happened, yet they had chosen to leave the subject alone.

The only comparable life event that impacted me so dramatically—aside from my brain surgery—and it was during a fragile stage—was when I became so agitated over standing in front of my class to give a speech that I had to leave the class for the day. My peers rooted for me from their seats, and it really was the only thing that helped me complete the course.

Similarly, Burke and Bender rooted me on in my distress, and I was able to push on. They went ahead that night to tease me about my dating life, or lack thereof, which made me think about Mary Grace, and share my insecurities with the guys.

"Just go for it!" Burke shouted. "You have nothing to lose!"

"Absolutely Nothing!" agreed Bender.

"Call the girl up and ask her out!" Burke laughed and threw a strike.

• • •

28
STEALTH

THE WAY Rex Stealth talked to me originally, part excited, part bored that I was interested in some freelance work, I kind of expected I wouldn't hear from Synergex again, even though Rex suggested a phone interview. He spent all kinds of time singing the company's praises, but even more time emphasizing individuality among it's employees, and he no doubt had already seen my extensive online profile, which listed experience to the contrary.

But he contacted me a third time, and asked that I come to an interview at my design school. It felt good to receive an invite, and it was nice to head back to my old stomping grounds as a leading candidate.

I spent the first half of the day catching up with professors and secretaries, checking out new artwork in the gallery, listening to the opinions of new attendees.

I was a bit taken aback when I wasn't the only interviewee; three other candidates sat around a long conference table in the green room, awaiting the same fate.

I had spoken to Terrence Pincher about my reservations concerning Stealth. Eternal optimist that she was, Pincher felt good about the upcoming interview. So much so, in fact, that she picked me up at my house, and offered to take me home after the meeting.

We all had our laptops and designs prepared for a presentation. The web designers were nervous, and us graphic designers were more seasoned. It made it interesting.

We all had been asked to create our own versions of a Synergex website and accompanying ad material. I wasn't that impressed by the two web designers, liked the second graphic designer's ideas, and thought I presented well, considering it wasn't my specialty.

Time would tell whether Stealth wanted to utilize my talents, to hire me. He made clear that he only had enough money to hire one person in the moment.

• • •

29
COURAGE

I MUST HAVE picked up my cell phone and placed it back on the orange recliner near my bed three or four times before I built up my courage enough to ask Mary Grace the question I had feared posing all my life.

My heart raced and my voice quivered whenever I practiced in front of my bureau mirror. I had given up hope that the sound of my voice would change, but I still clung to the possibility that I would experience a greater confidence.

The only thing that encouraged me was my imagination. I could hear Burke and Bender in my head urging me on, telling me I had nothing to lose and everything to gain. And, you know, I couldn't have agreed more.

Before trying again, I breathed deeply, ran my hands through my hair a couple times, looked straight into my reflection, and told myself repeatedly that I could do it. I tried to anticipate a positive response.

I wasn't the type to get rattled by little things. In fact, I prided myself on my strength. And yet this small act, this contact attempt, tested my willpower. Was I up to the challenge?

I called the doctor's office because I knew she'd be there working her tail off, picking up where the triage let up. Right this very minute she was probably standing between the automated double doors, fetching her next patient from the lobby. It took a while but I eventually got ahold of her.

She was breathing heavily when she put the phone to her ear. She said, "Mary Grace speaking . . ."

"Hey Mary Grace! Its Chris."

"Hi Chris."

"So listen . . . Uh . . . I was thinking maybe."

Silence. "You were thinking, huh?"

"Yeah. I was thinking, if you are up to it, that maybe we could go out together?" I crossed my fingers and winced.

"Are you asking me on a date, Chris?" I laughed uncomfortably.

"I guess I am."

. . .

EPILOGUE
PUSHING ON

IT WAS that time. The point when all leaguers had to say yes or no to another eleven weeks. After what I had gone through, I initially debated back and forth if I could even return to the alley.

But I had gone back, and I had pushed on. I had even salvaged my initial so-so average. After all was said and done, I could feel good about my accomplishments.

Over the speakers, Marge announced that she would stop at each lane and ask for commitments and contact information. I expressed to her beforehand that I was interested.

I patiently waited my turn. One by one, lane by lane, she took down names and numbers until she was finished.

Burke and Bender told me they intended to move on, that they had had their fill of bowling. That meant I had to find another set of teammates who wouldn't fear me, who could overlook the condition, and would accept me for me.

The thought was one that, at another time, would have crippled me. But as I followed after Marge, I had a good feeling about my new teammates. Marge had paired me well the first time, so I trusted she would do the same again.

She explained as we walked that the league would take a six-week break, that those who chose to return would begin again in May. She said she would use the break time to compile team arrangements, but for me, she had a specific person in mind.

"I think you'll like this guy. He's new to the league, but I've known him a while."

As soon as I saw him from behind I recognized him. His bald head glistened as it did at the coffee shop. Stone was minus his usual attire, the green apron and slacks, and he leaned on a nice bowling bag that replaced the usual broom, but he seemed more relaxed. He wasn't bound by the rules of the workplace. I could relate. The freedom to avoid professional mores was one of the perks of independent work.

I stepped down into the bowling area, and placed my hand on Stone's shoulder.

"Well, isn't this a surprise!"

• • •